TRAVIS—

Thanks for keeping me on my feet.

Kris Palmer

2011

ISBN 0-7414-6447-0

Printed in the United States of America

Published April 2011

INFINITY PUBLISHING
1094 New DeHaven Street, Suite 100
West Conshohocken, PA 19428-2713
Toll-free (877) BUY BOOK
Local Phone (610) 941-9999
Fax (610) 941-9959
Info@buybooksontheweb.com
www.buybooksontheweb.com

Dedicated to:

My Mother
Stella Mae Palmer

You recognized my gift for words and encouraged me to pursue a career in writing. When I thought the best part of my life was over, you showed me an avenue to take and gave my life purpose.

and
My Family

Table of Contents

"Dancing With An Elephant"

Having Parkinson's Disease is like dancing with an elephant. You can't stop dancing when you get tired. You have to keep dancing until the elephant gets tired.

By:
Sharon Baker Lyon

Acknowledgements

When I decided to write this book, I was unaware of the wildly emotional ride I was in for. I want to recognize those most instrumental in keeping me in balance, healthy and motivated while in this phase of the journey.

Mary Beth Lurk – My Sister
Emotions spilled forth from me as I relived difficult situations during the writing of this book. Mary, my precious other half, had the insight to put things in proper perspective and her calm nature grounded me. Without her, I may not have completed this project, which is of such importance.

Sandy Kossmann – Friend. You saw my pain and understood how deeply depressed I was. You threw me a lifeline called hope and helped lift the shroud of sadness in which I was cloaked.

Joanne Phillips – Poet, Published Author, Amateur Comedian. Your rousing personality and steadfast faith in my abilities kept me laughing and motivated when I needed it most. Without a doubt, you are my loudest cheerleader.

During the completion of this project, my friends enthusiastically stepped forward adding their expertise to mine. My manuscript was transformed into a polished work of art—a book that I am proud to have their creative fingerprints on.

Susan Haley – Award-Winning Novelist, Poet, Editor. Susan, as my editor, was adept at looking at my work with a fresh eye. Without changing my voice, she fine-tuned and tightened my writing lending it a clearer, more professional sound.

Linda Neckel-White – Accomplished Poet, Artist, Photographer. Linda formed the Voices of Venice poetry group. Under her direction, this amazing cluster of writers flourished, inspiring me with their talent and imagination. Linda's artistic background and eye for photography are evident by her design of the cover art on this book.

Sharon Baker Lyon – Poet. Sharon is a poet with an amazing gift for wrapping up a profound message in a few words. Sharon's keen insight enabled her to write the poem that ultimately became my book title.

Paula Knudsen – Queen of The Frumple Factory
Have a Frumple of a day! Be grateful, smile and play! Your dreams come true if you are true to them!
Paula's Contact Info: 941-685-0035
Frumples100@yahoo.com

Prologue

It began about fifteen years ago. Home on disability, I was feeling depressed and lost. I remember this thought going through my mind. I should write a book.

My ego argued with the voice saying such negative things as, What? You can't write! What could you possibly have to say that would interest a reader? You need a story, Kris. You don't have one. Regardless, I began journaling little by little.

As God would have it, I do have a story to tell. As the tale of my life and my path to understanding unfold, perhaps you'll feel a bit of kinship with me. Without exception, every human being will be challenged at some point in their life. If, through my personal experience, I am able to help just one person benefit, then my story is worth telling.

Preface

Dear Friend,

If you are reading this book, I offer you my hand in friendship. I sincerely hope that you will benefit from my experiences and that it gives you a sense of direction making a positive difference in your life as you move forward.

You're the only one that can do it, not your doctors, your significant other, nor me—only you. But that doesn't mean you're all alone. Accept the love and support offered you and share the glory with all.

A few years into my diagnosis my world got smaller. I could no longer hold down a job and quit working. I lost touch with my working friends. I lost touch with myself because all my roles had changed. I felt so sad at all my losses. I'm happy to say that has definitely changed today. My life is so much fuller and richer now than I ever imagined possible. I have met some of the most extraordinary people. They pass judgment on no one. Everyone is accepted exactly as they are.

We are all unique individuals at different places in our lives. We are all here to learn different lessons and our education comes to us in a variety of ways. Lessons are learned through positive, as well as negative experiences. There is no wrong or right way. We just are and we all serve a purpose.

Armed with this value system and feeling completely free to be who I am, has opened my eyes and my heart to infinite possibilities. I'm aware of my power and have regained control of it.

In my opinion, it is much easier to be open-minded about new things when dealing with an illness. I had so much to lose! I had so much to gain! It went against my nature to just sit back, accept the diagnosis I was given and let the progression happen. I wanted to get better and I know you do, too. You have to be ready, though.

In the beginning, I wasn't. Like an ostrich, I put my head in the sand and hid. I recall reading about how important nutrients are to the body and that B vitamins are good for the nervous system. I dismissed it. What I had couldn't be fixed with vitamins. The doctors said it was incurable so why bother?

Open your mind and accept that all things are possible. You're the one living with your ailment and you're the one that needs to believe you have the ability to do more. I realize now that no single healthcare practitioner has all the answers and it would be foolish to put my life in one person's hands alone. Active involvement in my own healing has become a must.

Build a team that works together for your common good. I see a great neurologist who truly listens, allowing me to take an active role in the care he provides. My acupuncture physician and massage therapist is expert at reading my body. His treatments are key in keeping me in balance where healing is most effective. My psychiatrist and psychologist work together in helping me manage anxiety so that I can live a life without fearful thoughts consuming me. The combined expertise of these healthcare providers gives me confidence that I am getting the best care I could hope for.

In the beginning, I never really understood what the term holistic medicine meant. Most remedies have limited effect when standing alone, but in combination with other approaches, big differences and changes for the good can be realized.

Good luck to you. If I can do it, so can you.

Kris Palmer

Before The Elephant

I was born in Missouri—the second child of eight. I have six brothers and one sister. I love my big family and wouldn't have it any other way. We arrived in the following order:

Dave, Kris, Jim, Dan, Bill,
Mary Beth, Tony, and Jerry.

It takes a lot to raise a family this size. Dad was the sole supporter while Mom stayed home raising kids and taking care of the house. My siblings and I had responsibilities, too. We all chipped in based on our ages. I helped Mom quite a bit with the babies. In fact, the last two boys, Tony and Jerry, I claim as my own.

We lost Dan in a car accident when he was nineteen. No matter how big a family is, the loss of a member is shattering. He is still missed today. No one can ever fill his shoes.

I loved school and always looked forward to summer vacation being over so I could get back in the classroom. I was an avid reader. I think I read most of the books in my school's library and always looked forward to visits from the book mobile that brought a variety of books from the county library.

During summer vacation, I read eight books a week. Mom would leave me at the library while she went grocery shopping. I would borrow four books on my card and four on my brother's card until the librarian caught on and fussed at me for breaking the rules. It broke my heart and I cried over it. Can you imagine doing such a thing to a child who simply craved to read? It would not have hurt anyone if she had turned the other cheek and pretended not to know what I was doing. I loved American History and read biographies of famous people like Dolly Madison and Abe Lincoln.

I wrote my first book in sixth grade. I clearly remember my teacher assigning it as the major class project of the school year. She told us to look around the room at our classmates because one of us might one day become a famous author. It seemed unlikely to me at the time, but now look! I still have that book—mom saved it for me. It is one of my most cherished possessions.

Besides reading I spent a lot of time outdoors hiking, bicycling, swimming, ice skating and more. I had almost enough brothers for a baseball team, so I learned to play that, too. In high school I was on the cheerleading squad.

After graduating I worked for several local businesses. Accounting and clerical positions were a good match for me. My dream had always been to get married, raise a family and work in St Louis for a Fortune 500 company. I got married but it didn't last.

When the marriage went up in smoke, I pursued the job and got hired. I loved it and did very well. The opportunities for promotion, pay and benefits were excellent. Little did I know what those benefits would mean to me in the future. I remarried but that union was also ill-fated except for the blessing of two children. Now my story begins . . .

The Diagnosis

Vibrant and attractive, I had the career, marriage and family I'd always dreamed of. Little did I know there was a dark storm cloud looming on the horizon that would soon sweep in and alter life as I knew it. I'm glad I didn't see it coming.

Our daughter, Danielle, arrived first. She was a perfect, petite little girl weighing just nineteen pounds on her first birthday. We called her Dani.

Son Caleb joined our family next. He was a big, healthy, robust baby boy. By the time he was four months old he weighed twenty-two pounds and I was stuffing him into a size two Toddler.

I began to notice a weakness in my left arm accompanied by a pins and a needles sensation. It ached and I just attributed it to carrying around a hefty baby boy. When he seemed to be too much to handle, there was always his dad, a grandma, aunt, uncle or friend around ready, willing and able to hold him for a while.

Gradually, I became aware that my left thumb had developed a tremor and would turn into my palm. Easy enough to hide from the public—but I knew something more serious was happening. I didn't go to the doctor for almost six months. I kept hoping it would go away of its own accord, but on a deeper level I knew I had a serious problem and I suspected it was Parkinson's Disease.

Finally, it was time to face the music. I found a neurologist in my insurance network and made an appointment. He confirmed my suspicions and sent me to Barnes Hospital's Movement Disorders Research Group for an extensive exam. They gave me a firm diagnosis of Young-Onset Parkinson's Disease. It was a pivotal life-changing moment that I'll never forget as long as I live.

I had been handed a life sentence of living with a neurological disorder, a progressive disabling old-person's disease for which there was no cure. I only had symptoms on my left side and was told with a little luck, I would never experience symptoms on my right side. The prognosis was a good ten years, maybe twenty, before more severe progression impaired my quality of life. I may or may not develop dementia, etc., etc., etc. I saw no luck in any of this.

My husband and I left the sterile, brightly-lit atmosphere of the hospital behind. Outside it was completely dreary and raining as was typical of a

February day in the Midwest. A bone-chilling wind whipped at my coat as we hurried to the car in silence. There were no words of comfort.

As far as I was concerned, this was as good as it was going to get. I had a chronic progressive disease for which there was no cure. My todays would always be better than my tomorrows. That was my bleak outlook—my acceptance of this horrible thing that was happening to me and my family.

Instead of calling it a day, I insisted on going back to the office. I wanted to tell my boss, co-workers, car-poolers and friends and get it over with. I told everybody I could that day and informed them that I never wanted it mentioned again. This disease was not going to control me. A shield, not unlike the Berlin Wall, rose up around me. This wasn't coping, this was full-blown denial.

I loved everything about my life. No way was I going to let this happen to me! But, it did. The tremor persisted and I learned to cross my arms in an attempt to stabilize my shaking arm with my steady one. I'd often put my left hand in my pocket or sit on it to hold it still. What a toll this took on me! It was so stressful trying to appear still and poised while my insides vibrated and my left arm wanted to flap like a chicken wing with a life of its own. I held myself so tightly in check, I was knotted up like a pretzel.

One of the worst symptoms was the brain fog. At one time, I was very sharp mentally. I knew exactly what I was doing at work and exactly where I had filed important documents. I could put my finger on anything almost instantly and knew the status of most accounts without looking. This is a crucial skill in the fast-paced I need this yesterday, corporate world. Then the fog rolled in. I felt slow like I was trying to operate underwater. My thought processes were interrupted and incomplete. Scientifically, my neurotransmitters were misfiring. The catch phrase was cognitive dysfunction. How I hated that!

I was so completely worn down and exhausted; I literally didn't know which way to turn. There was no daylight at the end of my tunnel—only darkness and despair. I was thirty-seven years old with a daughter that had just turned four and a one year old son. They were so young! They needed a lot of care—how would I manage all this? Life was my banana and then I slipped on the peel! When I fell, I fell hard, and my family went down with me. I slipped into a severe depression.

Lost

Lost in the wilderness of my mind
My sense of direction had forsaken me.
Tormented with thoughts of what I might find,
In the bleak future I saw before me.

Eyes blinking away unwanted tears,
My mind filled with dread.

Body vibrating—consumed with fear,
Desperate—hanging on by a thread.

The next few years were difficult, at best. By
the time the kids were in elementary and middle
school we decided to leave Missouri in search of a
new life. We settled in Florida. Sunshine, tropical
breezes and the Gulf of Mexico beckoned us.
Somehow we thought we could escape our
problems, but a geographic move doesn't fix what's
broken. Our problems moved with us.

A Life Sentence

Why do I have a movement disorder? Why do I have Parkinson's Disease? Why me?

These questions have literally tormented me since that fateful day when I was given the diagnosis. Every healthcare professional I saw asked me the same questions. Is there a history of Parkinson's in your family? Have you ever abused drugs? Did you hit your head? Well-meaning friends advised me to let it go. There was no need to agonize over something I'd probably never get an answer to; no one had the answer.

Eventually, I stopped stressing over it because I was smart enough to know this wasn't helping my situation. However, the desire to know never really went away. There were times when there was no stopping my mind. If the doctors didn't know what caused it, how could they possibly cure it?

One day I was given part of the answer. "Slow Down!" In order to hear and feel God, I needed to slow my pace. This was the beginning. It would bring me to the door, behind which, the rest of the mystery remained. Once I settled my racing thoughts and calmed my shaking body down, I knew more would be shown to me.

So, I slowed down. I rested my body and relaxed my mind through meditation. Then I realized I couldn't just sit and be still. I had to learn to move through life while carrying peace and tranquility within.

Now isn't that just ironic? Parkinson's forced me to slow down so that I could learn to move.

I learned to control the erratic movements of my body with my mind, but only to a degree. The fact remains that I have a physical ailment and when the dopamine levels in my brain drop too low, it rears its ugly head. When the dysfunction reveals itself, I need all the inner strength I can muster. At times, my power and determination are such that I feel I can conquer most anything.

Then again, some days my human frailty will be in the forefront, dragging me down and keeping me from the challenge. At these times, I pace and rant and rave until I'm crying and begging God for mercy. I simply get to the point where the inner turmoil is worse than the disease. Unable to deal with it on my own, my Higher Power gives me the relief I so desperately need.

When this happens, I experience the true meaning of gratitude. I have now come full circle. Gratitude is what was missing. To be grateful for all the blessings in my life is paramount with starting my day off on the right foot. Now my priorities are straight. My focus is directed toward doing what I can to become healthier.

Why do I have a movement disorder? Why do I have Parkinson's Disease? The answer to these questions will have to wait.

Orange

A brilliant blazing ball of Orange,
dropping from the sky,
gifts the world with color
before the daylight dies.

The fire and warmth of Orange
sets the world ablaze,
The sky, the clouds, the water—
Orange rides upon the waves.

Orange flows over me—
warming up my skin,
Its healing power consumes me
when I invite it in.

Orange melts away the stress
and mental noise I hear,
the goodness that is Orange
now occupies my sphere.

I surrender all I am
to Orange's wondrous energy
as I embrace the strength
its love is giving me;

The fortitude to face
whatever life may bring,
keep my faith, feel my joy,
allow my heart to sing.

The silence that surrounds
me as I sit and meditate,
is interrupted only
by the sounds the ocean makes.

My heartbeats match the rhythm
of the swelling of the surf,
Body, mind and spirit
become one with Mother Earth.

Peaceful and calm within—
my mind is quiet and clear.
The beauty of this space in time,
I cherish and hold dear.

For in this very moment,
there is peace within my heart,
I'll take this feeling with me,
and with it, never part.

With soulful eyes I watch
as Orange slowly slips away,
continuing on its journey
to the dawn of a new day.

The Impact of Fear

Fear is a horrible thing with which to live. Fear sucks the joy right out of life. Breathing becomes rapid and shallow causing heart palpitations and dizziness. Fear changes the body chemistry as it releases adrenaline. To the extreme, fear can trigger a panic attack. Over-time these rises in adrenaline can be very damaging to the immune system.

It started when I was very young, possibly the age of five. My dad wanted to keep us safe. He made sure we understood the dangers of lawn and farm machinery and cars. We were taught to distance ourselves from any equipment that was running. Being a timid child, I did not want to think about getting run over or caught in a piece of machinery. It terrified me.

My older brother, Davey, and I were walking down the one-lane dirt road that bordered our neighborhood. There was no real traffic on this road, just an occasional car or two driven by someone that lived nearby. It was relatively safe and we were allowed to be there.

On this particular day, a state highway department truck turned into the lane. He had his blade out and was cutting the grass and weeds growing alongside the road. I didn't realize this. My only thought was to keep from being run over so I hid in the foliage. It was quite tall. I crouched down in it and was easily hidden from view. Davey knew better. He plucked me out of the grass and off the road to a safe place.

I'll never forget how scared I was that day. I have carried that fear with me through my entire life adding to it, experience by experience, trauma by trauma, until I've developed an irrational fear of what could happen. From a very young age, I had fabricated fears based on what might happen, not necessarily on reality and I was still doing it.

This was a huge breakthrough for me on understanding and managing my fear. Now that I had an awareness of the fear I'd been harboring, my mind continued processing memories and thoughts. It was like watching a slide-show of my life experiences with fear. One by one as the memories arose, I released the fear associated with them.

Parkinson's Disease is an insidious thief. Dopamine producing cells are dying off for years before the first obvious symptom appears to the patient. By this time, most of these critical cells have been destroyed leaving the patient with a mere 20% that continue to function until, they too, die. It attacks the physical body robbing it of abilities once taken for granted. Crueler yet, it can plant paralyzing fear in the mind.

Some days are a struggle from the get-go. I cannot quiet my mind nor stop the racing thoughts stampeding through my head. I shake. I rattle. I roll. I scream. I rant. I rave. I cry. I beg. Above all, I ask, "Why? Why? Why?" Yet, it doesn't matter why. It is what it is.

Then, all the fears surface. I can't get behind the wheel of a car. What if I shake? I could lose my license. I might have a wreck. I drive too slowly in traffic. I might have to pull over. I'm on a bridge. What am I going to do? What in the HELL am I going to do?

Help me! Send me an angel! Help me! I talk to friends. I call my sister. I call my mom. I talk to God. I beg for help. I beg for mercy. I beg for death!

When this isn't happening to me, I love my life. I have all this potential that isn't being realized and I want to . . . I want to make a difference! I want to overcome this, and then, show others how to overcome it. I want peace, to feel safe, to live. I want to live!

It will all come with acceptance and I just don't know how to accept it. I don't! I keep thinking I can make this go away—I can make it better. I can do all the right things and heal myself, but the fact is that I can make myself healthier, but I can't take away Parkinson's Disease. I can't! It's not going anywhere! It's here and it's here to stay. How can I accept it? I just don't know. I don't know how to accept it.

I sweat. I blow snot. I'm giving up a lot of my social life and I don't feel attractive anymore. I'm just at my wits end! I hate this and I resent it. I have all these wonderful tools I've been given that help and I resent using them. I resent needing them. I take this resentment and internalize the anger. That's all I feel . . . the anger.

When I've finished carrying on, I stuff what's left inside because I don't know where to go with it. I put on a brave face and act like I'm in control of this, but I'm not. I can't control it and I hate the fact that I haven't risen above it. I want to so badly. I don't want this to be the focus of my life. I am more than Parkinson's Disease. I'm so much more.

Some days it's 2:00 p.m. and I still cannot get centered. The trembling goes on for hours at a time—days at a time. I know my mindset has a direct impact on how my body reacts. If I allow fear in, my self-talk becomes negative. "I can't stop this shaking! I hate this. God, take this away! I can't deal with it any longer! I'm tired of living this way. I'm scared."

I'd felt alone for so long. This, too, I internalized. Fear threatened to grip me and I struggled to control it. I didn't want others to know what was happening to me because I didn't think I could take it if I saw my fear reflected in their eyes. So I hid it to the best of my ability and wondered how much they saw. I was in a situation where I thought I would be disloyal to my partner if I admitted to myself just how unhappy I really was. The inability to be completely honest with myself and being separated from my family of origin kept me from reaching out for help. I stood alone.

Was I fearful that I wasn't worthy enough to ask for help? Was it pride and stubbornness that made me believe I could do this alone? Was it fear of failing and being exposed as such? Was I afraid of exposing my vulnerability and then going through the pain of disappointment? I had come to a point of desperation and often wondered how I could possibly go on like this.

Without consciously being aware of it, I had allowed fear to put limitations on me. In so doing, I'd quit experiencing so much that life has to offer. I'd built walls around myself, but they were beginning to crack. Fear was consuming me and threatening to take over. I could no longer hide behind it. I wanted my life back.

The years passed. Now teenagers, my children were on the threshold of making their own way in the world. It was a time of change. Unfortunately, never really having had, fully, the support of my husband, I stood alone then. And, I stand alone now but without the complications of a problematic marriage

Prayer and meditation were the avenues I took that finally brought me some relief. Once I asked God for help, it came in many different ways. In my case, the angels took care of my inability to speak for me. While listening to an inspirational lecture at a church service, I was overcome with emotion. Every word seemed like it was meant especially for me. By the time the speaker finished, I was weeping. Her words had touched my heart and told me that I was not alone. Out came a box of tissues and loving arms. I haven't stopped crying since and I hope I never do. Tears are a release I'd been denying myself for years.

Little by little, I opened up and shared my heart's desire to be healed. I asked friends, family, and members of my church to pray for me and send loving thoughts and energy my way. I am a child of God. I am made in His image. I am worthy. Taking the advice offered to me by so many, I visualized what I wanted and believed that it would manifest. Pulling in all my resources, I took back my power. Having opened my direct link to God, I was ready.

For years I desperately wanted, and still want, a cure for Parkinson's Disease. A miracle cure! What I wouldn't give to wake up tomorrow and have it gone. Just gone. I wanted my life handed back to me on a silver platter—no strings attached. My prayer was simply, "Please, cure me." I made it all about me and Spirit doesn't reward that kind of arrogance.

Gradually, I came to realize that I should consider bartering with Spirit. I decided to make a pact and changed my prayer. "God, if you will cure me, I promise you I will do something important with my life." I meant it, too! I put it out there . . . gave it to the Universe. I meditated on it and willed it to manifest but, still no cure. Looking back, I'm not surprised. I simply wasn't getting it.

A door of opportunity opened and I was invited to go on a spiritual retreat with several other women. What I remember most about the retreat was the joy that came bubbling up inside of me. Here I was amongst hundreds of people in deep prayer and contemplation; I felt so happy I wanted to laugh out loud.

Throughout the day, individuals gave testimonials regarding past healing experiences. One woman's story made a huge impact on me. Having been diagnosed with MS, she and her husband traveled to Brazil on a healing journey. She made a healing request and her first priority was that she learn to love herself without condition. Her second request was to be healed of MS. Her husband was confused. Had they journeyed all the way to Brazil just so she could learn how to love herself? What about the MS? She explained her belief that a cure would not be forthcoming unless she loved and nourished her body with good nutrition, adequate exercise, proper rest and positive self-talk. It was important that she embrace her illness and love herself in spite of it. Her prayer was answered. On the second trip to Brazil, she was healed of MS.

We are made in God's image—spiritually, emotionally and physically. We have the capacity to rise above our humanity and make great changes. Healing is a process in which all three aspects of our character, body, mind and spirit must be in harmony. I've learned that the power to heal is within me. I've been given the gifts of strength and courage to deal with life's challenges. It is my miracle. Having learned this, I once again changed my prayer. "God, I promise to do my best to fulfill your plan for me."

Acceptance Is a Process

I was so angry it was years before I could even consider acceptance of Parkinson's. I stubbornly refused. This was an intolerable situation and I carried my rage inside like a torch keeping the fires of anger burning.

I harbored worry inside because it allowed me to feel as though I was controlling an uncontrollable situation. An uncontrollable situation doesn't change because I worry about it. With worry, I ruminate and dwell on the same set of thoughts over and over. This doesn't prevent bad things from happening, but it does deter me from looking at the situation objectively. Once I identify and challenge my rationalizations to worry, then my ability to solve the problem at hand improves.

I didn't have the courage to take an honest inventory of my feelings. I stuffed negative emotions like fear and anger down with food. It only helped temporarily because I didn't get rid of them. They were simply buried under excess pounds that I had gained from overeating. This compromised my health even further, not to mention the damage it did to my self-esteem.

So, I worked on acceptance. But, I had it all wrong. I not only accepted it, I did a radical flip and embraced it. I became a Parkinsonian, building my identity around my disease. I had so much to learn about manifestation. Whatever I believed became my reality. I had basically given up and surrendered to PD; therefore, I got worse.

One of the most difficult things about living with PD is being alone with your thoughts. It is imperative to keep your mindset in the light because dark fearful thoughts can be more disabling than the disease itself. Does that mean thoughts are the disease? If so, then changing my thoughts can change the course of my whole future.

Thank God for the good people He puts in our paths. Beverly, a very gifted massage therapist, had been treating me for years and we had developed a deep friendship. She watched me decline and listened to me when I had one of many pity parties. I voiced over and over to her that I didn't want to live like this anymore. I was ready to die and leave this body of mine.

Bev minced no words. She had a heart-to-heart talk with me and pointed out that she couldn't help me until I decided I wanted to live. There were resources available to me but I had to use them. I had to do the work.

I knew she wanted only the best for me and so I listened. It was shocking to hear my words repeated back at me. I didn't mean them—they were really a plea for help. I wanted to live a full and productive life. It was a turning point.

Shaking and perspiring uncontrollably, Beverly suggested I go into a meditative state while on her treatment table. Breathing deeply, I relaxed and imagined myself at the summit of the mountain where my wise man resides. The air is crisp and cool here and I feel better already.

I found myself alone on the mountaintop. Where was my wise man? Just then, a jumbo jet silently floated by. It was so close I could see the passengers looking out their windows at me. Piloting the jet was my wise man! He was taking all those people to Heaven's Gate where they would speak with St. Peter.

Bev suggested I sit down in the wise man's chair while I think about what I'd just witnessed. I'd never seen my wise man sitting in a chair, so I began looking around for a nice smooth stone to sit on.

Suddenly, I found myself in the cockpit of a plane and I was in the pilot's seat. At Bev's prompt, I began describing what I saw. When I told her about the gauge indicating the horizon by which you align the wings and keep the plane level she wanted to know how I knew what that was. I explained that

I have an old friend who is a pilot. He'd taken me flying once and shown me how to use the gauge. It's not as easy as it looks!

The next thing I know, my wise man is sitting next to me in the co-pilot's seat. He's smiling and giving me non-verbal advice; he's communicating feelings, not words, telepathically. Just like the plane, I have to keep myself centered and in balance as I navigate my journey through life.

I was in crisis on Bev's table. I had given up on getting better and was letting Parkinson's Disease ravage my body. It was time for me to decide whether I wanted to live or die. My wise man was with me during this pivotal moment in my life. I wasn't alone. Loving energy knows no boundaries. My wise man reached across the physical dimension, touched my soul, and infused me with hope. I'll never forget it. I finally felt at peace.

That evening, I was ready to end my inner turmoil. First, I had to change my belief system. I learned that I didn't have to like or surrender to PD to accept it, but I did need to face reality and deal with it. Out with the negative thoughts and speech; I had no room for self-defeating behavior.

As I learned to listen to my body and give it what it needed, a sense of peace came over me. I directed my energy in a way that gave me more positive results. I experienced the total uncon-ditional acceptance of who I am in every way. It was a whole new approach to a way of being.

My True Colors

Pink! Oh my gosh! My beautiful champagne blonde hair had a pink cast to it! At least it was pink where the hair dye had taken; the rest had definite shades of gray. Just a few short years earlier, I had been proud to turn forty because I looked very young. Now, I was packing on thirty extra pounds, my breasts were too heavy to be considered perky and my hair was pink and gray!

Something had to be done, but what? I couldn't reverse the aging process and I didn't have the funds, or the desire, for cosmetic surgery. I didn't even want to pay a professional to color my hair. Besides, hadn't I always said that beauty comes from within?

Acceptance! That was the key. I decided to go one step further and embrace the aging process. If I was going to pull this off, I knew the first thing I needed to change was my attitude. In this materialistic world, where we idolize youth and the teenage girl's body, we are setting ourselves up for so much unhappiness. A teenage girl's body is not fully developed. If we try to look that way for the rest of our lives, we are denying ourselves what we need to be healthy and strong.

The chiropractor that I was seeing suggested I quit coloring my hair because the chemicals in the hair dye would sit on my scalp while processing and leech into my brain where they couldn't escape. This painted quite a vivid picture of the toxins I was voluntarily feeding to my brain and that's all it took.

I set out on an adventure. I decided to let my hair grow out to its natural color and see what I had. I was actually curious. This was easy for me to do because we'd recently relocated from Missouri to Florida. As it was, if the results were not flattering, I wouldn't be seen by anyone who knew me.

I took a good long look at the reality of what I was dealing with and knew that it had no significance. Whether I was a blonde, a brunette, a redhead or gray would make absolutely no difference in who I am. Armed with this knowledge, my attitude quickly changed.

I had enough physical problems without contributing to them for the sake of beauty. Beauty is in the eye of the beholder and I decided to be a beautiful, middle-aged woman and go gray gracefully. That is exactly what I manifested. To my delight, the hair that framed my face was a beautiful shade of silver.

Then, the most remarkable things began happening. Complete strangers began to comment on how pretty my hair was. Numerous women said they admired my courage and wished they were brave enough to show their true colors.

I'd gotten more than I'd bargained for. I had gracefully accepted the color of my hair and all the connotations that go with it. I learned a powerful lesson in this acceptance, and as a result, I gained admiration and respect. People really began to see the beauty and strength within me and admired my courage to proudly stand alone.

I Stand

I stand before the mirror,
perplexed by what I see.
I don't remember growing older.
Is this really me?

I look closer . . . study the map of my face,
Each line represents a path
that led to this place.
Some are laugh lines,
others riverbeds of my tears,
tension, from hurry and worry through the years.
Melded with these lines are smooth areas of peace,
signifying goodness in my life,
rapture within reach.
My life is full of purpose—

rich with people that I love.
Gratitude is what I feel,
for these blessings from above.

Aging is a fact of life. It's part of the path I walk.
Acceptance is all important.
This is not idle talk.
Superficial beauty, may fade
with time as I grow old,
be replaced with wisdom
as life continues to unfold.

I stand before the mirror,
at peace with who I am . . .
A beautiful, mature, wise woman,
I like the skin I'm in.

Love Your Tremor

A wise woman once said to me,
"Love your tremor and all it can teach you."
Outraged, I did not quite understand
what good that could possibly do.
This was a lesson in self-love
that I desperately needed to learn.
If I hated the Parkinson's tremor,
at myself, the anger would turn.

I embraced my tremor, it is part of me,
I changed my attitude.
This took time—it didn't happen overnight,
But, eventually, I felt gratitude.
Realizing that God loves and accepts me
In spite of any imperfection,
Taught me to love and accept myself
as I am, without condition.

On-Off Syndrome

With Parkinson's Disease there is a phenomena called "On-Off" syndrome. When "On" the body is working efficiently enabling it to function in a nearly normal state. When the medication wears "Off," dysfunction reappears.

On-Off. On-Off. On-Off. This goes on all day long. Every three hours I am scheduled to take my prescription medications. I really try to be consistent and take them on time, but sometimes remembering completely escapes me. I forget.

When I feel well, my focus is on anything but PD. A vibration or a leg cramp, any one of a number of symptoms shows up to remind me that it's still there. I must feed the elephant and keep it at bay. I cannot stress enough how important it is to give the body what it needs to function properly.

I have my tool chest to rely on. My tool chest contains a list of things to try that may alleviate my symptoms. This includes certain foods like bananas which are high in potassium, or cucumbers and celery which help cool my body if I'm feeling warm. Calcium and magnesium aid in easing the cramps in my legs and feet. Stretching exercises and yoga are very effective in maintaining balance and good posture. Deep breathing exercises have a calming effect. Sometimes I need a change in my environment, so, I take a walk and focus on the birds and wildlife.

I am fortunate enough to live just five minutes from a beach. The sound of the surf is so soothing and, of course, the view is breathtaking. A phone call to a friend gets my mind on other things. Journaling is an excellent way to vent my frustrations and get to the core issue of what may be bothering me emotionally.

Seldom do I know what it is I need. It's a matter of trial and error. So I try different things at random until I find one that gives me some relief. If nothing works, then time inevitably takes care of it for me. The three-hour cycle begins again with taking my prescription meds.

Acts that are simple to perform when I'm functioning well can be difficult and time consuming when I'm not. Sometimes they become impossible to do at all. For instance, when getting dressed, bras and socks really challenge me. Fine motor skills and flexibility are needed here—a constant reminder to continue exercising.

When eating, unless there is a sticky placemat that grips my plate, cutting my food is difficult at best. The tremor actually pushes the plate around on the table causing me to chase after it. The only solution is to surrender and try again in a few moments. I've learned to do this. It wasn't easy and took quite a while because I was so headstrong. I'd hang in there and push my way through, but it made the tremors worse. Now I know it's best to stop for a moment, take a deep breath, regroup and try again.

Many days, I appear far more normal than I feel. Sometimes I feel under stimulated and trapped inside of myself. I'll sit for hours and obsess with playing games on the computer just because it's mindless, doesn't take much effort.

Everyday tasks can take so much time and energy when dealing with a tremor and slow thought processes. At other times, I feel over stimulated and overwhelmed. My mind will race with thoughts of everything I have to do but I can't seem to grasp what is most important. Unfocused, I'll literally walk from room to room, doing a little here, a little there and not accomplishing much of anything.

I had a particularly difficult morning today. There really was nothing unusual about it except for the realization that came to me. Aggravated with myself, I thought it pretty sad that I couldn't hold my focus long enough to complete a ten minute task. With a newfound clarity, I realized my neurotransmitters were misfiring. My brain couldn't complete a thought; therefore, my body couldn't complete an action. I tell myself, this is not my fault; I am not losing my mind. I have a physical ailment.

The first step is to acknowledge what is happening and let go of the anger and frustration with myself. By looking at the bright side, I allow myself to take a break and just enjoy the stillness. I've learned to just be with it and accept it for what it is. It's only temporary; it always stops after a while. I hang onto that thought and ride it out. After all, I succeeded in leaving PD behind when I stepped on the golf course. So I decided to go to the golf course in my mind. I decided to walk in my mind when my feet cramped. Never again would this disease stop me. Never again!

In the past, I'd rage against myself because of these limitations. Misguided anger certainly didn't help. Now I was opened up to an awareness of what was really going on in my body enabling me to address that issue in a proactive way. The next step was to see what I could do to jumpstart my brain into functioning. What was even possible?

I began by asking myself questions and trying things until I'd find something that helped. Every day and every situation required different action. PD certainly keeps me questioning my needs because they change from day to day, hour to hour. The one common factor is to keep moving—physically and mentally. I push myself. Even though a certain amount of downtime is necessary, I have to be careful not to become too sedentary.

I've learned not to berate myself for downtime. I've always been a doer. I'd snatch ten minutes waiting in line at the grocery store to read a paperback book. I seldom watched a movie or TV without doing something else with my hands like counted cross stitch or embroidery. PD ended that. It was no easy task for me to learn to focus on just one thing. I felt like I was wasting time.

How do I deal with the issue of wasted time? I feel that God is giving me the opportunity to slow down for a reason. I certainly don't think I would have done so without being forced. He shows me the way toward a more peaceful, less hurried existence. Still, my brain resists with a strength and intensity that is amazingly powerful. If I can learn to channel that in a more positive way, it will contribute greatly to my healing.

When I am "On" and I feel like my old self, Parkinson's Disease couldn't be further from my mind. That is the blessing in all of this.

Lost For Words

Choked with emotion—
I find it hard to speak.
My legs are uncontrollable,
they feel so weak.

I know that I can't stand still;
I'd have to march in place.
I know that I can't sit still;
I'd have to jump up and pace.

I feel oh so restless—
full of nervous energy.
I wait for the medication to work
and create some synergy.

Soon I'll feel a wave of relief,
wash away my pain,
As everything begins working
and my abilities are regained.

The most precious Gift from God
that I receive each day
is when the tide brings in good health,
and I can break away.

Commitment

It takes a conscious decision and a dedicated commitment to set a goal and pursue it. Perhaps, the most important virtue needed is patience. As Americans we are in such a hurry to get there that we sabotage our own efforts by not allowing enough time to reach our goals. We want our rewards and we wanted them yesterday. It took me a while to accept the fact that I needed to make life-style changes. These take persistence . . . slow, steady, consistent steps in a forward direction.

Bill, acupuncture physician and massage therapist, is also my friend. As such, he took it upon himself to give me some guidance in starting and establishing an exercise program. He encouraged me to swim daily but I continually procrastinated and came back with excuses for not doing so. One day, frustrated with hearing yet another excuse, Bill looked me in the eye and said, "Kris, you just don't want to do it." The truth in his words hit me like a brick wall. I opened my mouth to defend myself but found I could not. He was right.

What I had just heard wasn't anything new to me. What was new was the realization that I'd been lying to myself. Wow! Now I had to take a good hard look in the mirror. If I was lying to myself in this situation, how many other lies had I believed? Instead of just admitting the truth, my subconscious mind was intent on keeping me from it by fabricating some ridiculous untruth that I actually believed. I lived by it.

This is amazing. I was shooting holes in my own plan to do whatever it takes to become healthier. It's now time to reflect on my past and see if I can remember when this all began.

I have made a commitment to myself to do whatever it takes to become healthier and I will not be swayed. I am on a healing journey that is bringing me results I haven't dared hope to achieve. I am training my body to function appropriately.

I've been on the fence the last few years, not really buying into the fact that I have the power to make living with PD whatever I believe it to be. Now that I understand, I'm actually looking forward to the future. I have a more positive attitude and; therefore, I will get more productive results. I feel hopeful and challenged. This is exciting! I can heal. I may not be cured, but I can definitely heal. The progress I've made so far really excites me. To know that I've turned this thing around and I'm winning the war is so encouraging. I've done the hardest part. I can keep trekking forward now and watch the miracles unfold.

Remember, this is critical, move at your own pace. Wherever you are is where you need to be and only you will know where that is.

What I have come to realize is that nothing is set in stone. Nothing! That includes Parkinson's Disease and how it will progress and affect me. Just because the doctors say it is so doesn't mean it is so. If I change my mind, I will change my life.

I choose to set my mind free to explore. The Universe is vast and there is no limit to the possibilities available to me. Every day I have the choice to see the world as a playground full of promises. Nothing is impossible, until I believe it to be so. I choose which life I want to create, who I want to become. I focus on it without wavering. I believe in myself.

Over the Fence

Leaning against the fence
Indecision driving me mad,
Staying here stuck in the past
Playing it safe, can be terribly sad.

Sitting on the fence
In gratitude for this safe space
All's well in this moment called *Now*
Can't stay . . . the future has a new face.

Jumping over the fence,
Anticipation catching my breath,
Giving up fear for a life that I love,
Living it . . . no regret.

The Warrior

The truth is, I find myself going along my merry way and then a tremor appears out of nowhere. That's all it is, just a tremor. If I can stay in that mindset where the truth lies, then it simply remains what it is, a Parkinson's tremor. But, if I allow fearful thoughts to dominate, the tremor becomes colossal. It transforms into an unrecognizable beast that can consume and cripple simply by invading my thoughts. It is a mind game that manifests in the physical.

I knew I had to transform from the timid, trembling person I was into a vital warrior fighting for my life against an enemy of my own creation! Taking on the persona of a warrior, I became strength, courage and determination. The moment I adopted the spirit of the warrior, I saw all the things that were standing between me and victory. I vowed to fight and win.

The next day my doubts and fears would return with a vengeance. I'd ask myself, "How many times must I slay this beast?" The answer . . . as many times as it takes.

Bill shared with me this piece of wisdom. When in the midst of trembling, I can use this. Give myself permission to sit back and just let it be. I've been fighting to control the tremors and I just can't do it! They'll subside when my elephant tires of the dance.

The Kris that used to be an open book is no longer the girl she was. She has embodied the Spirit of the Warrior. With integrity, she will protect and love herself first. Only then, will she have the ability to regain her strength and live into her full potential. I have taken back my power.

I was in awe. With clarity I can only describe as holy, I understood. I was the only one in charge here—no one else, just me. I also understood that I was the only one who could fulfill my dream of perfect health and also the only one that could cause my failure. This is not meant to understate the importance of support from caregivers, friends and loved ones; but, it's me who decides when to call upon them.

Inspiration spread through me, warming my cold hopelessness. I was getting my life back—just like I had prayed for.

Discouraged

When I feel discouraged and want to quit,
I say a prayer of thanks
for these trials that are a gift.
Inside the challenges I face, are riches galore,
Treasures of inner fortitude, perseverance . . .
and so much more.

Believe In Yourself

Believe in yourself and you can do anything.
The only thing stopping you is you,
so, step out of your way and greet this fine day,
with positive intentions and your best.

Believe in yourself,
others will believe in you.
As they see you embrace your personal power,
what began as a quest to do your personal best,
may inspire others to put themselves to the test.

Believe in yourself and watch the magic spread.
Keep your eye on the future—keep moving ahead.
As you realize your dreams and they come true,
the life you create has a beautiful view.

Don't Get Caught With
Your Pants Down

Courage is the ability to step out of your comfort zone and move through your fear. People tell me I'm brave—that I have courage. I agree my life is challenging at times, but I don't exactly consider myself brave. A survivor is more befitting.

Most people do not see me during my "off" periods when the neurotransmitters in my brain are misfiring and command signals are interrupted. I'm reduced to shaking, perspiring and talking to myself. I've had to actually coach myself through a series of movements just to get out of bed. It was either that or lay there crying.

Try to imagine not being able to roll over, sit and get out of bed. These moves were learned as an infant and can be done automatically by most, but it is no easy task for someone with cognitive dysfunction. It takes thought, planning, and a rocking motion to get started. It also helps to count each step as it aids the smooth flow of movement.

One event illustrates a giant step forward in this part of my journey through the battlefield.

For more than fifteen years, I've been having hot flashes. They have steadily gotten worse. Today, I can only describe them as extreme. They come on with a vengeance and last for hours. Just this morning, I had a flash that lasted about an hour and fifteen minutes. This evening I endured another three hours. In fact, it's not unusual to suffer six or more total hours in a day.

These are not what I consider normal hot flashes. I have never had one at night. Never have I awakened to soaked pajamas and sheets. I can't tell you how many years it has been since I had a flash that came and went in ten to fifteen minutes, perhaps never. When they finally abate, I feel very cold. It's as though my body has an inability to regulate its temperature.

What is causing this to happen? I have to know so that I can get some relief. Is it due to monthly fluctuations of hormone levels? Is my thyroid the culprit? Are they side effects of my medications? Are hot flashes caused by anxiety, or does the hot flash bring the anxiety on? Which comes first? It's the old chicken or the egg dilemma. Nobody has the answer, but I refuse to accept that. I know that Parkinson's will become easier to manage if this problem gets eliminated.

In retrospect, I call it my, don't get caught with your pants down theory. Looking back, I'm able to see the humor in every situation . . .

How on earth was I going to get out of this predicament? I had dressed too warm this morning. Being from the Midwest, I still was not accustomed to how quickly a cool morning could turn warm here in Florida. I should have worn shorts. Once I began feeling warm, I knew I had about ten minutes before I was thrown into a hot flash which would affect my weakest link, Parkinson's Disease. Not wanting to drive while in this condition, I stopped at the park to take a walk and settle down.

The sun was intensely hot. My jeans were sticking to me from all the perspiration running down my torso and legs. There wasn't a dry spot on me. I needed to sit in the car and run the air conditioner on high until I cooled down, but another problem presented itself. I had to go to the bathroom and I had to go now!

It was all I could do to manage peeling my damp jeans down far enough to empty my bladder. My underwear came down in one tight roll. I had avoided an embarrassing accident! Relief washed over me but it was short lived when I realized that I had an even bigger issue now.

The park bathroom was stifling hot and I needed to get outside where the air was moving. Even a hot breeze would feel better than this. I managed to pull my underwear up, but my jeans were stuck and I was getting more desperate by the minute.

Then the door opened and in walked a woman dressed in the green uniform worn by park employees. I was so glad to see her. If she had sprouted angel wings right then and there I would not have been surprised. I explained my situation and asked her to help me. Without a word, she grabbed the center belt loop on the back of my pants and gave it a good yank. She literally shook me back into my jeans as though she was stuffing a pillow into a pillow case. I thanked her profusely as she turned to leave. She acted as though it was all in a day's work, but to me it was much, much more. I hope a copy of this book finds its way into her hands one day and she recognizes herself because I want her to know how much I appreciate her kind act of mercy.

Be prepared, for the unexpected, and don't get caught with your pants down! This experience planted a new seed in me. Definitely out of my comfort zone, I was forced by a situation to reach out and trust again.

The difference in me today is that I'm smarter. Before I give my trust away, I look into the eyes, the windows to the soul, and I listen to my instincts. I recognize an abuser when one crosses my path. I immediately set boundaries and do not allow him or her into my realm. This was and is hard for me because I want to believe in the basic goodness of people.

Evil always disguises itself as good. This is what makes it so difficult to discern. Proud of their strength and power they have no remorse for their actions. One must develop an acute awareness of their environment. Keep your eyes wide open and see the truth.

The most successful evil doers are very good at hiding their true selves. They reveal whom they are when they are ready. It is imperative to surround yourself with the right people. Choose individuals that inspire and support you in bringing out your best.

My world had closed in on me and gotten smaller. I had limited myself. Now, I had to reach deep inside and grab the desire to change and do something with it. I decided to start with breaking a habit that was not serving me.

Breaking a habit begins with awareness and an intense desire to change. The inclination to drop my head and look at the floor is always there. Focusing on correct posture and resisting the urge to curl forward can be a real challenge because my head is used to falling forward. That is now my comfort zone. I have to push past that zone to hold my head high.

My resistance is so strong that it sometimes triggers severe tremors. I've learned to push myself to the brink and when the tremors begin, stop, and be with them for a moment, then back off just enough to return to a point of stillness. Each time I work on breaking this habit, I go a little farther stretching my comfort zone. This is an essential part of my recovery.

Now that I could hold my head high for a longer period of time, I worked on improving my eyesight. Since I spent most of my time at the computer, reading a book and doing housework, my long distance vision had really suffered. I began spending more time outdoors. As I walked, I looked out into my environment and focused on objects at a distance. I also did some eye exercises that strengthened and sharpened my vision.

I am determined and certainly won't give up without a fight. Perhaps, I do have courage, after all.

The Lion and The Lamb

Here I am, trembling again.
Let my guard down and your memory slipped in.
Now I'm frustrated, tied up in knots,
Shaken, bent over . . . I'm seeing spots.

My heart is heavy with the humiliation I bear
from years of being treated like I wasn't there.
Like a defeated, weak and fragile old soul . . .
this woman I've become, I don't want to know.

This weakness of Spirit, I cannot abide.
I pull from the strength I have deep inside.
I take a full breath, and stand up straight.
I'm better than this; I won't be afraid.

Shoulders square and head held high,
I remind myself that the limit's the sky.
I can do anything I set my mind to.
Nothing will stop me—not even you!

For, I am a person in my own right,
True to myself, I move into the light.
It's here I discover who I really am . . .
Strong as a lion, yet, meek as a lamb.

Exercise

My friend, Bill, is such a phenomenal coach. He knows I listen to and respect what he has to say. He is never judgmental or condescending; only professional, persistent and patient. Without his treatments, guidance and friendship I know I would not be nearly as well as I am today.

To quote Bill, "Move that body!" He meant it, too. Move! Do something every day. I used to believe there wasn't much point in exercising because I couldn't do the workout of a trained athlete. But that doesn't mean I can't do my very best from the place I'm in. All I need to do is move at my own pace. The key is to set small goals and have reasonable expectations. Once I reach my goal, I then set another target and keep moving in a forward direction. I am amazed at how far this has brought me.

Being one that needs to see measurable results to stay motivated, I chart my progress. I keep this simple. For each day that I exercise, I color in that block on my calendar. This gives me a very visual display of what's been achieved by week and month. I supplement my diet and exercise regimen with vitamins and herbs. For each bottle emptied, I give myself a pat on the back. The empties are tossed in a box and when it is full the amount of good fed to my body looks back at me. My reward is a resounding "Yahoo" as I acknowledge the change in how I feel and function. It becomes readily apparent that baby steps do make a difference.

My re-entry into the world of movement began on the golf course. Bill took me along to watch him play. Immediately, I loved the game and being on the course; it reminded me of my home state of Missouri. My psyche was starved for green grass, open space, shade and cool breezes. Time seemed to stand still while on the course. I felt so relaxed . . . actually soothed. It was a wonderful escape from the fast paced noisy world that Parkinson's is at odds with.

Weak and insecure, riding in the cart was all I could manage the first year. One day I idly mentioned that I would like to learn to play golf. Bill put a putter in my hand and I was hooked. That Christmas he gave me a set of clubs and I've been playing ever since.

The game of golf is perfect therapy for me. It takes intensive focus and flexibility. I learned to find that moment of stillness between tremors and swing the club. Sometimes after swinging the club, I was left standing and shaking but I had managed to make contact and set the ball sailing. What a triumph! Through sheer determination, I had pulled that drive through the eye of a needle. I did it again and again. Each time it became a little easier to find and stay in that moment of stillness.

There's no competition between Bill and me, only camaraderie and acceptance. My only competition is within me; the warrior versus the elephant. With Bill I just play the game and very seldom keep score. Each stroke is new; we don't worry about how we played on the previous hole. We have fun and that brings joy into a life that had, for too long, become burdensome to me.

The changes in my fitness level and state of health are amazing. Within two years, I've progressed from simply riding in the golf cart to playing the game while walking the course and pulling my clubs behind me. All this, seventeen years into the disease when many people suffer more severe impairment as Parkinson's progresses. What's not to be thankful for?

After winning my battle on the golf course, I started going to the swimming pool five days a week or more. I have always loved the water but now I feared it a little. I felt stiff and ill at ease. Staying motivated was a challenge because I've been caught in the pool when my meds wore off and it was very uncomfortable. I stayed with it. Some days all I could manage was to get in the pool, get back out, and go home.

Swimming, like anything new and unfamiliar to my body, tends to hit a trigger catapulting me into wild tremors and weak knees. One day, I literally hung on the side of the pool in the deep end close to an hour, too weak-kneed to even think of climbing out. Someone asked me if I could swim—that's how obviously uncomfortable I looked.

After that experience, I started alternating the times I went swimming to further challenge myself. Sometimes I was alone in the water. At other times, it was crowded in the pool. Both situations presented different issues to deal with.

I admit it was stressful and many times I didn't actually get any exercise to speak of. But I held fast and didn't quit. I kept going through the motions and before I knew it I was beginning to swim. I added in some water aerobics and increased my swimming to laps. My strength increased and my muscles became toned.

After about two months, I got a sign that my efforts were paying off. One day my left arm was trembling and felt real stiff, like a block of wood. But, when I swam, it relaxed and functioned in a normal manner. As soon as I stopped swimming, it resumed trembling. I had taught myself to move beyond Parkinson's to a healthier state of being. I was rebuilding neuro-pathways!

Incorporate exercise into your daily life. My advice is to stretch several times throughout the day to keep moving as freely as possible. I stretch before I get out of bed in the morning and again before I go to sleep at night. Stretch even when you think you cannot; such as when you have dystonia in your feet. Be gentle with yourself so as not to cause an injury. I watch an exercise DVD and follow along while sitting in a chair. Most stretches can be modified to work for you.

Find something that challenges you, something you enjoy, or it will become just another chore. Work out at the gym, walk, golf, swim, float, or sit in the shallow water. Do what you can. Start at your own level and give up being afraid of looking foolish. Conjure up the carefree person inside of you. Think, act, feel what it was like to be a kid and learn to have fun again. Enjoy taking a nap; it's a luxury most cannot afford. Read, play cards, bake cookies, or take a math class. The brain responds well to exercise, too. Do what you can. It may not seem like much at first but the rewards are there if you work at it.

My ego gets the best of me at times; after all, I am human. Some days I just don't want to exercise and instead of pushing myself I give in and don't do much of anything. One day turns into four or five and one morning I'll wake up barely able to move. I pay the price.

Move your body. Move your mind. Every day do something good for yourself that you enjoy.

Consistency will pay off and you will reap the rewards of perseverance. Don't be hard on yourself if you start out slow. Remember, baby steps make progress, too.

Move

Move that body, girl!
You're just collecting dust.
Move your mind and think.
To survive, it is a must.
When you take some action.
You immediately feel empowered.
Life takes on new meaning;
depression lifts as clouds.
Add a spring to your step
As your outlook takes a positive turn.
Reverse the aging process:
Reach for what you yearn.

Ninety Days

Ninety days or so, I guess it's been
Since I committed to a daily swim.
It has become a habit, much to my surprise.
I really like it—it sure opened my eyes.
I haven't always put forth the necessary effort
To adopt a new way of being.

By not giving it my best,
how could I ever know
What experiencing my goal could mean?
Benefits? I'm stronger, physically, I find
The most amazing change is in my mind
I have come to know, that I have a lot of power
In creating and living a life that's better by the hour.

The Mental Dance

I thought I had overcome feeling nervous, but it wasn't that easy. Anxiety, many days, was nipping at my heels. It took a great deal of composure to ignore the negative thoughts that threatened my peace.

I was on the golf course when it hit me. We were playing the first hole and there was a bottleneck. Four golfers were ahead of us and several behind. We were paired with two other players and I was waiting to tee off.

This is the beauty of the game of golf. It can teach us patience. I have plenty of patience and am relaxed and at ease when waiting for others. Put the shoe on the other foot, and I can get myself completely stressed out.

For instance, no one was waiting for me at the golf course. We were all waiting for each other as the game ensued but I had myself convinced that I would be to blame if anyone got impatient.

I was aware of what was happening, but I felt powerless to control it. My body began to shake and my breathing became shallow. Looking to Bill, I cried "I don't know what to do!" he said to me "choose." I chose to relax, let it go and enjoy the game.

Feeling rushed or knowing that someone may be waiting for me has been a stressor for me as long as I can remember. Being in such a situation, or even anticipating that I'll be late, really pushes my buttons. How do I react? Stuff the real emotion and start shaking.

When I realized that I had fabricated this stressor in my busy brain, it went away. There was no longer any reason to believe it was real. I could actually feel the physical release as it lifted off my chest.

Swimming, another of my great loves, can strike fear in my heart. I love being in the water but, I resist going to the pool. Why? Oh, I can dream up any number of excuses. I don't want to deal with a wet bathing suit or the chance that I'll get the shakes. I don't want to walk back with my foot twisting or drive back with my leg shaking. It's too hot. It's too cool. It's too windy. The truth is I'm afraid I'll get a cramp while in the pool and I don't want to be seen hobbling around when I get out. I don't want to take the chance that I may have to crawl over to a lounge chair.

Why do I let these things mushroom and grow so huge in my mind that they keep me from doing what I love? Even if I find myself in a bad space while at the pool, I know what to do. Just get in the water and float. The water will take it from me. But, oh no, my busy brain is working overtime. Somebody might be watching. What if somebody is looking? I have all my life worried about how I appear to other people. I never felt like I fit in so I always had to be perfect. I had to be pretty. I had to be together. I was silent because I didn't want to open my mouth and say something stupid. I didn't speak for fear. I let fear rule me—fear and worrying about my inadequacies. Oh, my goodness! It's time to stop this.

In reality, most people aren't looking at me anyway. So why am I so self-conscious? This morning I was up at the pool and some guy came in and swam. I don't even know if he saw me there and if he did it didn't matter because he was minding his own business. He left and I'm not even sure when he left but the whole time I was wondering to myself, where he was. What is he doing? He's not swimming anymore. Is he looking at me? That's ridiculous. Get over yourself, Kris.

Every day I spend time getting reacquainted with myself. I was watching a football game on TV and saw a shot of the cheerleaders. I was a bit surprised at my strong emotional reaction. Suddenly, I felt as though I was falling backward in time to when I was a cheerleader myself. Usually I think of my squad mates and I remember what our uniforms looked like. Not this time! I felt like a time traveler who was once again sixteen years old. I felt her! I recalled how much I loved cheerleading and everything that went along with it. Practices, games, pep rallies, parades, cheerleading camp . . . I was physically active in those days clearly because I loved what I was doing. I realize I've found that same passion today in playing golf.

I had so much self-confidence back then. Whatever I wanted I went after and got. There was no question about it. I figured out the steps needed to reach my dream and then I walked the walk and talked the talk. I was living my dreams because I believed in them.

In order to triumph over my illness, I had to change my approach and recapture that same youthful drive. I took it slow and steady. Change is a process. I opened my eyes and really looked at the world around me and how I saw myself fitting into it. I became aware of my environment and the natural order of things. I realized there was no need to hurry to get where I thought I needed to be because I was already there. If there was something that I wanted, I learned to be patient because I knew it would be waiting for me.

I learned to go with the flow—it's much easier that way. Once I finally accepted that the only thing I could control was me, I realized that was the simplest solution of all. In fact, it's the only way to live in true harmony. Trying to change the world to fit into my life only created more chaos.

I've been stretching and opening up and it feels so good, too. But every action brings with it a consequence. After years of constricting, my body rebelled at being pushed beyond its comfort zone and reacted by shaking severely. It was the type of episode that really challenged me mentally until I broke through to the other side. Heaven, it was. At the moment of perfect stillness, I was left with nothing but peace. I'd just had a taste of the Divine. I was enrolled for life. I'd never give up the fight now for I had tasted its rewards.

You tweak it and tweak it and tweak it until you find something that works and when you do, enjoy the flow because you're in it. You will fall out occasionally, and when you do, pick yourself up and get back in balance. Try again. Repeated challenges sculpt what you are in stone. That's the mental dance.

The Eye of a Storm

It's taking everything I've got
to stay calm while pen is to paper.
Emotions come to the surface,
making the challenge that much greater.

My legs are weak and quivering,
drawing up in one big cramp.
From my toes to the pain in my hips,
nothing, quite prepares one for this.

I want you to know what it's like
to live in the eye of a storm.
Where the mind is quiet and still,
In the midst of chaos all around

For in that stillness is peace
like you can't imagine but should know.
That's the place where you find yourself;
that's the place where your mind's in control.

Curb Service With a Smile

Dystonia is a lack of normal muscle tone due to disease of the nervous system. It is characterized by prolonged, repetitive muscle contractions that may cause twisting or jerking movements of the body or a body part.

Dystonia first appeared in the big toe on my left foot. Several doctors commented on it before I was diagnosed with Parkinson's. In fact, it was so slight I couldn't feel it even after they told me it was there.

It came on gradually over the years eventually getting to the point where my foot was relaxed except for my big toe pointing straight up. This strained the tendons in the arch of my foot causing a burning pain.

Pain is a human experience. No one gets through life without it. Pain manifests in many different ways. Some people suffer with physical pain or illness. Others deal with emotional pain; such as a family estrangement, death of a loved one, a failed marriage and, of course, the pain and frustration of dealing with chronic health issues.

The rest of my toes began to curl under as though I was making a tight fist with each foot. This certainly kept me off my feet and put an end to my early morning walks. That's when I got serious about swimming. One door closes and another opens.

For many more years, dystonia was a minor annoyance, but now it has become disabling. When my feet touch the floor in the morning, I've got about ten minutes before dystonia usually strikes. I can never predict how severe it will be, how long it will last, or if I will experience it on one side or both. When it strikes on both sides, it is even more unpredictable because it may move from one side to the other or affect left and right simultaneously. This is obviously the most difficult to work with. If caught on my feet when it strikes on both sides, I have little choice other than to get down and crawl.

Oddly enough, it helps to crawl. There's something about changing my position or pattern of movement that temporarily relieves the dystonia giving me the ability to get up and walk about ten or twelve paces to the nearest chair where I can safely get off my feet. The possibility of a fall or injury looms large, so I use forethought and planning before making any moves. Once seated, I massage my legs and feet and use deep breathing exercises to relax.

Eventually, I get to the point where I can get up and move about. I balance myself by lightly touching my fingertips to the kitchen countertop. I put all my weight on my steadiest foot while standing as tall and posture perfect as possible. This enables me to stretch out the cramped and twisted muscle on my free leg. Stretching while properly aligning the bones, tendons and muscle tissue does much to prevent dystonia and shorten its life span. That contributes to having a good day.

Sunday morning is my favorite time of the week. People are at church, sleeping in, or having a family breakfast. The neighborhood is quiet. There's no one out and about except for an occasional lone walker. This is my personal time to exercise, connect with nature, and speak with God. I cherish the solitude.

On Sunday mornings, I usually drive to the club house because it is gentler on my feet than walking. I take a swim and then sit poolside journaling while in meditation. I give my sore feet and legs a nice soak in the hot tub. From pool, to deck chair, to hot tub are all short distances I know I can traverse.

This particular day, there was a chill in the air, so I opted for a walk instead of a swim. For some reason, I felt infallible and it didn't even cross my mind that I could possibly have a problem finishing my walk and getting back home.

Enjoying myself, I reached the club house and walked around the perimeter of the vacant parking lot, when I suddenly felt the toes on both feet curling under. This spelled trouble. I couldn't possibly walk home like that, nor could I make my way to the club house. Sadly, I had miscalculated my abilities. Without any forewarning, I found myself in a precarious position, immobilized by clawed feet. Frozen in place, I looked around for a helping hand. I was completely alone with only bird song and the drone of a distant plane to keep me company.

I knelt down and worshipped God in his outdoor church completely prepared to crawl and walk, crawl and walk, until I made my way home. Surprisingly, I wasn't upset at all—I could do this. Taking one last look around and listening with a keen ear, I was convinced there was no one about. I placed my hands on the pavement and began to crawl.

Seemingly out of nowhere, a white car silently pulled up alongside me. I didn't see or hear it coming. I just became aware of a tire next to me and a concerned elderly couple asking if I was all right. They thought I had fallen down. I explained my situation and they offered to give me a lift home, which I gratefully accepted.

I never really was alone that morning. I believe God answered my prayer for help. He sent me two angels in a white car and provided curb service with a smile.

Life Interrupted

My morning was planned—some exercise, a shower and then on to my day. If I've learned nothing else, it's that things don't always go as planned, so it's best to remain flexible.

Step 2, 3, 4 . . . Step 2, 3, 4 . . . Step 2, 3 . . . When exercising, it helps to hear a voice giving me direction so I become my own personal coach. I've got cadence. I use the tempo and rhythmic sound of my voice to move fluidly. I opened my space, coached myself and marched indoors.

I lengthened my stride and swung my arms. When I reached the wall I froze, stopped right in my tracks! Weird, my natural ability to turn was gone. Like a malfunctioning computer, my short-circuited brain was valiantly searching for a connection while I hung out within myself feeling the sparks fly. I managed to turn by pivoting on one foot and pedaling around in a circle with the other.

My meds were due to wear off and I wanted to be showered, dressed and settled with a book before that happened. I showered quickly, leaving the door open because I was feeling claustrophobic. As I stepped out of the shower, my legs and feet were seized by very strong cramps.

No problem. I knelt on the bath mat and placed my palms on the tile floor. From this position I could pull with my arms and I'd slide effortlessly along on the mat. This was quicker than crawling and much easier on my knees.

There was one big hitch in my plan. The bath mat was soaking wet from keeping the shower door open and it didn't budge under my weight. Crawling was my next option but I couldn't lift either knee off the wet mat. Frozen in place, my arms began shaking with fatigue. My body was seized by a huge painful cramp. I was home alone.

Feeling my anxiety increasing, I began pulling in air in short shallow gasps. I screamed for help, but no one heard. Eventually, I managed to move about twelve inches, just far enough to reach the pocket door on the closet and slide it open. I turned over the laundry basket I found and braced my arms on it raising myself to a kneeling position. Exhausted, I could go no farther. I longed to lie down on the cool tile floor but was afraid I'd find myself in an impossible predicament. If I stayed where I was at least I'd remain closer to standing up.

Eventually, I surrendered and lay down. Immediately I felt some relief. The floor was cool and eased my anxiety. Also, the change in position relieved the muscle cramps. Saying a heartfelt prayer of gratitude, it was only minutes before I was back on my feet. The whole episode lasted about forty-five minutes but it changed me forever. I know that no matter how impossible a situation may seem, with time, it will change.

Sticks and Stones

Sticks and stones . . . While on the floor I had panicked because my inner voice was telling me I could not get up. They were just words but my fear gave them power. Who said words cannot harm you? For example, I detest the word incurable. It's just a word, a label given to Parkinson's Disease because the cure has not yet been forthcoming. For too many years, I lived with *incurable*. I was robotic—going through the motions like so many others robbed of hope, trying to accept their fate. How depressing is that?

Incurable is a word that causes so much fear through the ripple effect. I may not be able to strike it from the dictionary, but I can strike it from my vocabulary. If a word like incurable is in any way diminishing my sense of well-being, I eliminate it from my realm. If I should hear it spoken or see it in print, I give it a push as it flows by and replace it with a positive thought such as *I Am Well*.

Give it what it needs and the body knows how to heal itself. We've all been touched by something—broken bones, sprains, cuts, fever, or the common cold and our bodies have healed with the proper support and care.

There is a cure for Parkinson's. It begins with finding any deficiency in the body that is contributing to or causing dopamine-producing cells to die off, and then treating that deficiency. Researchers believe they are close to finding the cure. This knowledge is my driving force and supports my sense of well-being.

Retaining my independence is everything to me. Through my fear, I felt it slipping away that day. It's ironic, but it was this same fear that fueled my desire to live a full and productive life and renewed my conviction to make it happen. It's not an easy path, but I will be okay. I won't, CAN'T, take no for an answer.

Noise

I've been so aware of the noise this week!

First, I met Debby. She was very sweet; I liked her immediately. She talked almost non-stop for hours about a million different things. Although I found her very entertaining, I was literally tired after spending time with her.

Camille, the hairdresser, was next. A constant monologue poured from her. I sat back and relaxed, there wasn't room for me to speak anyway. Camille barely paused for air. I remember thinking as she cut my hair that I wouldn't trade places with her for anything! She was running in overdrive.

Two young moms with four children under the ages of six or seven were at the pool. Normally content to have the place to myself, I found my solitude invaded by high excited kid energy. These moms were on high-vigilance while their kids played like puppies in the water.

Then it hit me! I wasn't unlike these busy people I had encountered. The only difference was that they continued to feed the thoughts racing through their busy brains by verbalizing them. On the other hand, I used to internalize most of my thoughts so as to appear quiet.

Being conscious of the intensity of the noise going on in other people's lives made me keenly aware of the fact that my mind was quieter. With a smile on my face, I realized I had achieved a measure of the peace and serenity I was seeking.

Commotion

Words, phrases, melodies . . .
Stuff running through my brain.
Thoughts jumbled up and scattered
like a derailed train.
Bits of conversations,
memories I recall,
fears and worries I create,
illusions are they all?
Playing a song in my mind,
over and over again.
Can't shut it up, or turn it off.
Am I going insane?

Blended Healthcare

Having lived with Parkinson's Disease for close to two decades has given me real insight into the healthcare field and how it works. I was brought up believing that Western Medicine was the most advanced and therefore, provided more opportune care. Without the use of *Sinemet*, the most common drug used to treat Parkinson's tremors, I hate to think of what condition I might be in today. Still I believe that no one thing is better than another. It's the combination of therapies that makes an overall difference.

Without a doubt, I am extremely grateful for the benefits I've received from Western Medicine, but research and development move too slow for me. I don't have time to wait on the medical community, pharmaceutical companies, and politicians to muddle through all the red tape created by beaurocracy to find a cure. I have to take care of this myself and I have to do it now! This is my life. No one else has a bigger stake in it.

I turned to Eastern Medicine because its approach to illness is to strengthen the body and mind in order to resist the effects of disease. It's all about balancing life's elements to support healing. All aspects of these three categories; physical, mental and spiritual are treated.

Oriental Medicine has so impressed me. I'm sure a good part of that comes from the fact that Bill and I discuss everything about my condition; including how I'm feeling emotionally before beginning an acupuncture treatment. By addressing my fears and concerns, I am better able to relax and allow the needles to do their work. As the energy channels in my body are unblocked and opened to flow freely, I drift off to sleep.

Upon awakening, I feel very calm and composed. The treatment continues to process for a few days. Changes in how I feel overall may be subtle at first and then one day, I'll experience the *Wow Factor*. This is the sudden realization that my elephant has distanced himself. He'll be back, I know, but in the meantime I feel great!

Blending the best of both types of medicine is a powerful approach to treatment, which is similar to the way hospitals in China have been operating for decades.

Years ago, I went to physical therapy and learned a variety of exercises to remain as flexible, strong and mobile as possible. I've always been

home is pleasing to the eye and surrounded by beauty. It radiates with warmth.

I simply can't say enough about relationships and their importance. The sense of security I get from knowing my family is there for me is immeasurable. Growing up, Dad made it very clear that my brothers were to watch my back. They did then and still do today.

I have the "best" friends. I consider them my extended family. They are so endearing to me. Each one is special with unique qualities all their own. With personalities as different as day and night, my circle of friends brings variety into my life. Each one is a complete joy to me as I am inspired by how much they care. Without exception, my friends love me. Through them I have learned to love myself.

My circle of friends and family members care about and want to see me live powerfully. Just knowing I have their support gives me strength.

Home Is My Haven

My home is my haven; I set my standards high.
Within, only peace and harmony reside.
Family, friends and others I allow into my sphere
Nourish my independence, even as I hold them near.
I strive to stay in balance, steady and calm
by keeping my thoughts positive,
using love as a balm.
All of this good energy permeates my home.
Here I can relax and know, I'm always safe from harm.

What Comes Next?

Well, I've made it this far. What comes next?
I've been moving ahead in faith, step by step.
Diligent, it seems as though progress is slow.
   Until I look back, and see how I've grown.

I take it one day at a time—sometimes less.
   Break it down into manageable slices;
Anything worth having takes effort and time.
To reach the top of the mountain, one must climb.

   And climb and rest . . . climb and rest
The sky is the limit—I put myself to the test.
   One foot forward and then the next.
Keep moving ahead—it's not that complex.

When I reached the summit—I came to realize
   As I looked around, with a satisfied eye
   I had reached my goal,
Yet, there's room to achieve before I touch the sky.

Epilogue

As a result of walking such a challenging path, I've become a person that I like and respect. Parkinson's Disease came to me bearing Gifts of courage, patience and compassion. Above all, I have adopted a spirit of determination and refuse to take "no" for an answer.

There is nothing pretty about Parkinson's but there is a beauty that comes from living with it. It's the reward of knowing what truly matters, and living life accordingly.

Those of us with Young-Onset Parkinson's Disease are struggling to remain a viable part of society. Many of us have young families and are still raising children. In spite of our cognitive difficulties, our minds are bright. We refuse to sit back and watch life pass us by. So we work our minds and bodies to maintain our vitality. Life's simple pleasures bring a new meaning to the experience of absolute joy.

Please join me in advocating support of the cure for Parkinson's Disease and all other neurological disorders. Let our voices be heard. We will not be forgotten!

Kris Palmer